NAVIGATING SPONDYLOLISTHESIS WITH CONFIDENCE AND CARE

Empower Yourself With In-Depth Insights And Proven Strategies For Bone And Spine Recovery

DR. WESLEY IAN

DISCLAIMER

The information in this book is not meant to replace professional medical advice, diagnosis, or treatment; rather, it is meant mainly for general informational reasons. If you have any questions about a medical problem, you should always consult your doctor or another trained health expert. Don't ever discount expert medical advice or put off getting it because of something you've read in this book.

Any negative effects or repercussions arising from the usage of the material provided herein are not the responsibility of the book's author or publisher. It should be noted by readers that the material in this book is not all-inclusive and might not address every facet of the subject. Furthermore, new research may have an impact on how health concerns are understood or treated because medical knowledge is always changing.

No particular test, treatment, method, or product mentioned in this book is endorsed or promoted by the author or publisher. The reader assumes all risk associated with using the information included in this book.

Before making any big decisions regarding your health, it's crucial to speak with a licensed healthcare provider. The relationship between a patient and their healthcare practitioner should not be replaced by this book, nor is it meant to offer medical advice.

The opinions presented in this book are the author's and may not necessarily represent those of the publisher. Any errors, omissions, or inaccuracies in the information in this book are not the responsibility of the author or publisher.

It is recommended that readers independently confirm any information contained in this book and speak with a healthcare provider about their specific medical needs and state of health.

TABLE OF CONTENTS

ABOUT THE BOOK

The invaluable book "Navigating Spondylolisthesis with Confidence and Care" tackles the difficulties of having spondylolisthesis and provides a thorough manual for comprehending, treating, and living well with this spine ailment. The book starts with a comprehensive introduction that gives readers a general understanding of spondylolisthesis, its various forms, and the particular function it fulfills. Information clarity also goes a long way toward defining the intended readership, explaining who stands to gain the most from the insights offered in these pages.

The basic elements of spondylolisthesis are explored, including its definition, forms, causes, risk factors, and common symptoms. This basis gives readers a firm comprehension and paves the way for the next investigation into the effects of spondylolisthesis on day-to-day functioning. An in-depth analysis of the effects on mobility, emotional health, employment, and day-to-day activities is provided in Chapter 2, which presents a comprehensive view of the illness that goes beyond its physical effects to encompass its psychological cost.

The book offers a road map for understanding spondylolisthesis medicine. Different medical strategies for treating the illness are explained. Treatment choices, drugs, pain relief, physical therapy, rehabilitation, and surgery are all covered. The book deftly shifts its focus to self-care tactics, including helpful guidance on exercise regimens, lifestyle decisions, ergonomics, stress management, and the critical role that enough sleep plays in controlling spondylolisthesis.

The book's exploration of gaining confidence in day-to-day tasks is one of its most distinctive features. The author offers empowering ways to overcome obstacles related to spondylolisthesis, ranging from managing job and profession to interacting with others, forming relationships, and participating in outdoor activities. The value of support networks and resources is emphasized. It is acknowledged that a holistic and resilient attitude to living with spondylolisthesis can be fostered by friends, family, support groups, communities, medical experts, and educational materials.

"Navigating Spondylolisthesis with Confidence and Care" essentially serves as a source of empowerment and knowledge for those who are dealing with this illness. Its methodical approach guarantees that readers will have a comprehensive arsenal for managing spondylolisthesis in their daily lives, starting with knowing the fundamentals and progressing to self-care techniques and confidence development. The book encourages readers to be resilient and self-assured in the face of the difficulties presented by spondylolisthesis in addition to providing education.

CHAPTER ONE

INTRODUCTION TO SPONDYLOLISTHESIS

KNOWLEDGE OF SPONDYLOLISTHESIS

A spinal disorder called spondylolisthesis causes one vertebra to slide ahead of the other, usually in the lumbar (lower back) area. This illness can cause varied degrees of discomfort and disability, which can lower someone's quality of life in general. Investigating spondylolisthesis's definition, kinds, causes, risk factors, typical symptoms, and diagnostic techniques is crucial to understanding the condition's complexity.

It is necessary to investigate the structural consequences of spondylolisthesis inside the spine to define it. The name comes from the Greek terms "olisthesis," which means slippage, and "spondylos," which means vertebra. Spondylolisthesis, which compromises the integrity of the spine, is essentially the forward or backward displacement of one vertebra relative to the next vertebra. The several types of spondylolisthesis seen in clinical settings may be caused by this displacement, which could be the outcome of several underlying causes.

TYPES AND DEFINITION

Based on the origin and cause of the spinal dislocation, spondylolisthesis is classified. Isthmic and degenerative spondylolisthesis are the two main kinds. A deformity or fracture in the pars interarticularis, a short bone section linking the facet joints, is frequently linked to isthmic spondylolisthesis. Conversely, age-related changes such as disc degeneration and facet joint inflammation frequently result in degenerative spondylolisthesis. Because each type exhibits distinct traits, diagnosis and treatment must be customized.

REASONS AND DANGER ELEMENTS

Clinicians and patients alike must have a thorough understanding of the causes and risk factors associated with spondylolisthesis. While degenerative spondylolisthesis is primarily connected with aging and related structural degradation, isthmic spondylolisthesis can be attributed to genetic predispositions, recurrent stress, or traumatic accidents. Risk factors are a wide range of factors that can affect an individual's susceptibility to acquiring this spinal ailment. These factors include age, gender, genetics, and lifestyle choices.

TYPICAL SYMPTOMS

A person's everyday life may be greatly impacted by a variety of typical symptoms that frequently accompany the appearance of spondylolisthesis. These symptoms can include tightness in the muscles, decreased movement, and pain spreading down the legs (sciatica). The degree of spinal dislocation and the existence of nerve compression affect how severe the symptoms are. Understanding these signs is essential for prompt action and efficient spondylolisthesis care.

METHODS OF DIAGNOSIS

The use of diagnostic techniques is essential for both verifying the existence of spondylolisthesis and identifying its particular features. Imaging tests, including computed tomography (CT) scans, magnetic resonance imaging (MRI), and X-rays, are essential for determining the degree of vertebral dislocation and for displaying the structure of the spine. A complete medical history, physical examination, and neurological assessment also help medical practitioners gain a thorough understanding of the patient's condition, which informs the creation of a treatment plan that is appropriate for the patient.

Spondylolisthesis is a complex spinal condition that necessitates a detailed comprehension of its definition, types, causes, risk factors, typical symptoms, and diagnostic techniques. Healthcare providers must have this thorough understanding to accurately identify patients and provide individualized treatment plans, which will eventually improve the health and quality of life for those who are impacted by this illness.

CHAPTER TWO

COMPREHENDING THE EFFECT ON EVERYDAY LIFE

IMPACTS ON FLEXIBILITY AND MOBILITY

Technology's pervasiveness in our daily lives has had a big impact on our freedom and mobility. People now have more mobility because of the introduction of ride-sharing services, GPS apps, and intelligent transportation systems. The ease with which a ride can be requested with a few smartphone clicks has changed the nature of traditional transportation. Concurrently, more flexibility has been made possible by remote work arrangements, which let people work from almost anywhere. People's daily routines have changed as a result of this transition, leading to a lifestyle that is more flexible and dynamic.

MENTAL AND EMOTIONAL HEALTH

Technology's effects on mental and emotional health are complex phenomena. Social media offers forums for communication, support, and expression, on the one hand. On the other hand, anxiety and feelings of inadequacy might result from frequent exposure to carefully chosen content and the need to maintain an online identity.

Furthermore, the widespread use of cell phones and their continual connectivity may be a factor in increased stress and digital exhaustion. Positively, several online resources and apps for mental health include methods for stress management, emotional support, and mindfulness, highlighting the dual impact of technology on mental and emotional health.

EFFECT ON DAILY ACTIVITIES AND WORK

Workplace technology integration has completely changed how people work and go about their daily lives. The introduction of collaboration platforms, automation, and digital communication tools has improved efficiency and streamlined procedures. Technology has made remote employment increasingly common, making it harder to distinguish between business and personal life.

Although there are benefits to this flexibility, such as better work-life balance, there are drawbacks as well, like the possibility of burnout and trouble setting boundaries.

People's use of technology has changed the way they interact with one another, manage their time, and do business on a personal and professional level.

ADAPTING TO CHANGES IN LIFESTYLE

People's lifestyles have had to shift due to the rapid advancement of technology, and they are constantly adjusting to these changes. Adopting new technology while being aware of its possible drawbacks is part of adapting to lifestyle changes.

It takes deliberate decision-making to strike a balance between the advantages and disadvantages of technology. Some strategies include establishing digital boundaries, using technology with awareness, and combining offline activities.

It also entails keeping up with new developments in technology and how they could affect people's day-to-day lives so that people can choose wisely how to incorporate these innovations into their daily lives. While coping mechanisms can take many forms, understanding how technology is changing will help you navigate the changes it brings.

CHAPTER THREE

TREATMENTS FOR SPONDYLOLISTHESIS MEDICALLY

One vertebra being displaced over another is known as spondylolisthesis, a spinal disorder that frequently results in pain, stiffness, and neurological problems. Spondylolisthesis is treated using a multimodal strategy that takes into account the patient's unique characteristics, the degree of spinal displacement, and the intensity of symptoms. In this section, we discuss the several medical techniques for treating spondylolisthesis, including medication, physical therapy, and surgery, as well as the significance of customizing a treatment plan for each patient's particular situation.

AN OVERVIEW OF AVAILABLE THERAPIES

Relieving symptoms, enhancing the general quality of life, and improving spinal stability are the main objectives of spondylolisthesis treatment. Options for treatment can be generally divided into two categories: surgical and conservative methods. Conservative approaches are frequently the first to be tried, but in more serious situations or when conservative approaches are insufficient, surgical treatments may be taken into consideration.

DRUGS AND PAIN CONTROL

The use of medications is essential for spondylolisthesis pain relief and inflammation reduction. Pain and inflammation are routinely managed with the prescription of nonsteroidal anti-inflammatory medications (NSAIDs). Given that spondylolisthesis frequently results in muscle spasms, prescribing muscle relaxants may be advised. While there are situations where short-term usage of opioid drugs may be justified, their long-term effectiveness and potential for dependence need to be carefully examined.

In addition, analgesic drugs, such as acetaminophen, can be used to treat pain. To maximize outcomes, a holistic strategy for pain management frequently combines prescription drugs, physical therapy, and lifestyle changes.

REHABILITATION AND PHYSICAL THERAPY

A key component of conservative care for spondylolisthesis is physical therapy. The goals of therapeutic exercises are to increase total spinal stability, strengthen core muscles, and increase flexibility.

Physical therapists collaborate closely with patients to create specialized workout plans that target particular imbalances or weaknesses that are aggravating the disease.

To reduce discomfort and increase joint mobility, manual therapy methods like massage and manipulation may also be a part of rehabilitation regimens. Long-term success depends on educating patients about ergonomics and good body mechanics, which will enable them to take an active role in their healing.

PROCEDURES SURGICAL

When non-surgical treatments are ineffective or the spondylolisthesis is severe and linked to neurological impairments, surgery may be considered. Spinal fusion, which attempts to fix the afflicted vertebrae, and decompression surgery, which relieves pressure on the spinal nerves, are common surgical procedures. Improvements in surgical techniques, like minimally invasive procedures, help to shorten recovery periods and provide better results.

The choice to have surgery is very personal and is based on a careful assessment of the patient's preferences, lifestyle, and general health. A thorough evaluation of the possible advantages and dangers of surgery is conducted, with the patient actively participating in the process.

SELECTING THE APPROPRIATE COURSE OF THERAPY

A thorough evaluation of the patient's health and preferences is necessary to determine the best course of treatment for spondylolisthesis. The decision-making process for therapy is guided by various factors, including the degree of spinal dislocation, the existence of neurological symptoms, and the impact on everyday functioning. A multidisciplinary approach including neurosurgeons, physical therapists, orthopedic surgeons, and pain experts guarantees a comprehensive assessment and customized treatment strategy.

A variety of techniques, from conservative therapy to surgical interventions, are used in the medical care of spondylolisthesis. To optimize outcomes and enhance the overall quality of life for people with spondylolisthesis, choosing the best treatment strategy requires careful consideration of each patient's unique characteristics.

CHAPTER FOUR

SELF-MANAGEMENT TECHNIQUES

EXERCISE AND STRETCHING ROUTINES

The cornerstones of a healthy lifestyle are regular exercise and stretching regimens. In addition to helping one maintain a healthy weight, physical activity is essential for improving one's flexibility, strength, and cardiovascular health. A comprehensive approach to fitness is ensured by partaking in a range of exercises, including strength training, flexibility training, and aerobic workouts. Exercise is enhanced by stretching practices because they increase the range of motion, promote flexibility, and guard against injuries. These practices, whether they involve an organized exercise program or just basic daily stretches, help to improve mental health, lower stress levels in the muscles, and boost energy levels.

Sustaining a Healthy Lifestyle: Sustaining a healthy lifestyle entails making deliberate decisions that support mental and physical health. This includes consuming a healthy, well-balanced diet, drinking plenty of water, and abstaining from dangerous behaviors like smoking and binge drinking. Regular health check-ups, screenings, and preventive actions to address any health issues proactively are also part of a healthy lifestyle. People can strengthen their immune systems, increase their vitality, and lower their chance of developing chronic illnesses by cultivating healthy habits, which will provide the groundwork for a happy and active life.

POSTURE AND ERGONOMICS

It is impossible to overestimate the importance of good posture and ergonomics in day-to-day tasks. Preventing musculoskeletal problems and encouraging comfort and efficiency are critical goals of ergonomics, the science of designing settings to fit the individual. Whether standing or sitting at a desk, maintaining proper posture lowers the risk of back and neck pain and supports spinal health. Long-term physical health and discomfort prevention require implementing ergonomic concepts into workspaces, selecting supportive furniture, and paying attention to body alignment during different activities.

TAKING CARE OF STRESS AND MENTAL HEALTH

In today's hectic environment, taking care of stress and giving mental health priority is essential to general well-being. Deep breathing exercises, mindfulness meditation, and taking up hobbies are examples of stress management practices that can greatly reduce the effects of stressors. Mental resilience is influenced by creating a solid support network, getting professional assistance when necessary, and cultivating wholesome connections. People can maintain a healthy and meaningful existence by actively addressing stressors and acknowledging the significance of mental health.

The importance of getting enough good sleep is paramount to overall health and well-being. Sleep is essential for several physiological functions, such as immunological response, mental clarity, and emotional stability. Improved sleep hygiene is a result of establishing a regular sleep schedule, making a cozy sleeping environment, and kicking disturbing habits. Making getting enough sleep a priority not only helps with physical healing but also with mental clarity, emotional stability, and general resilience in the face of daily obstacles. It is crucial to acknowledge that sleep is a non-negotiable aspect of self-care to support a balanced and healthful way of living.

CHAPTER FIVE

INCREASING SELF-ASSURANCE IN EVERYDAY TASKS

MANAGING YOUR CAREER AND WORK

Gaining confidence in day-to-day tasks is essential for both personal development and general well-being. In managing one's work and career, for example, confidence is a major factor. Confidence affects not just one's performance but also one's perception by superiors and coworkers in a work environment. Establishing specific objectives, learning necessary abilities, and producing high-quality work regularly are crucial elements in developing confidence in the workplace. Strong self-assurance in the workplace can also be further enhanced by accepting setbacks and seeing them as chances for improvement.

RELATIONSHIPS AND SOCIALIZING

Building meaningful relationships and interacting with others is another area of daily living where confidence is essential. Being able to interact with people in social or professional contexts demands a certain amount of confidence. Developing excellent communication techniques, active listening skills, and a sincere interest in other people are all necessary for boosting confidence in social circumstances.

People can develop enduring relationships and progressively increase their social confidence by venturing beyond their comfort zone and participating in social activities.

TRAVELING AND ENGAGING IN OUTDOOR ACTIVITIES

Engaging in outdoor sports and travel offers additional avenues for enhancing self-assurance. A sense of success can be gained from venturing into unknown territories, attempting novel experiences, and welcoming adventure. Resilience and self-reliance are fostered when travel-related obstacles are overcome, such as navigating foreign places or trying new activities.

These encounters not only widen perspectives but also provide a basis of self-assurance that transcends ordinary life.

OVERCOMING OBSTACLES WITH SELF-BELIEF

Furthermore, the idea of confidently conquering obstacles is essential to personal growth. Obstacles are an inevitable part of life, and how people handle these problems often says a lot about their confidence. Overcoming hurdles with confidence is largely dependent on cultivating a growth mentality, in which setbacks are seen as chances to grow and learn.

Seeking assistance from others, establishing reasonable objectives, and acknowledging minor accomplishments during the journey all contribute to a resilient and optimistic outlook.

To sum up, developing confidence in day-to-day tasks requires a comprehensive strategy that takes into account many facets of life.

A person can become more self-assured and resilient through navigating their job and career, interacting with others and building relationships, traveling, participating in outdoor activities, and conquering obstacles. Through proactive efforts in these domains, people can boost their confidence, resulting in a more satisfying and prosperous existence.

CHAPTER SIX

RESOURCES AND SUPPORT SYSTEMS

FAMILY AND FRIENDS

A person's general well-being greatly depends on their family and friends' support system. These intimate bonds frequently act as the cornerstone of emotional support by giving people a feeling of security and belonging.

The relationships that are forged between friends and family members constitute a network that can provide support, empathy, and consolation during trying times.

The ability of a person to cope and get through challenges can be greatly impacted by the support of loved ones, whether they are dealing with personal troubles, health issues, or life upheavals. The reciprocal character of friendships and family relationships—where people can assist one another and feel interconnected—is what makes them so strong.

COMMUNITIES & SUPPORT GROUPS

Support communities and groups, in addition to the immediate family and friends, are essential in giving those facing particular issues specialized help and understanding. These organizations bring together people who deal with issues related to mental health, navigating life transitions, or coping with illnesses in common. Support groups provide a safe space where people may talk candidly about their difficulties, exchange coping mechanisms, and show understanding for one another. These networks help people feel less alone by fostering a sense of camaraderie that can accompany particular life circumstances. Support groups, whether they are held in person or virtually, provide a forum for people to get consolation and inspiration from people who genuinely understand their particular circumstances.

HEALTHCARE PROFESSIONALS

Whether a person is experiencing medical or mental health concerns, healthcare professionals—such as physicians, nurses, therapists, and counselors—are an essential source of support. These experts offer knowledge, direction, and a methodical approach to dealing with health issues. The foundation of the connection between patients and healthcare providers is communication, trust, and a commitment to promote well-being. In addition to providing medical care, healthcare professionals can also be sources of knowledge, instruction, and emotional support. Their responsibilities go beyond providing medical care; they also include maintaining patients' health and working together to obtain the best possible outcomes for their health.

OBTAINING EDUCATIONAL RESOURCES AND MATERIALS

In an information-driven age, having access to educational resources and materials is crucial for those who want to comprehend and deal with a variety of issues. By providing people with information about their problems, available therapies, and support networks, educational materials can empower people.

Information transmission, whether via books, articles on the internet, or instructional initiatives, is a tool for empowerment. Getting access to resources might involve more than just medical knowledge; it can also involve advice on coping mechanisms, lifestyle modifications, and community programs that are offered. Educational resources support people in taking an active role in their well-being and aid in making well-informed decisions. Furthermore, the availability of services promotes a cooperative approach to support and care by helping caregivers and support networks recognize and assist individuals in need.

EMERGING TREATMENTS

New and creative approaches to treating a range of medical disorders, including spondylolisthesis, have been made possible by recent advances in medical research. Regarding spinal problems, new treatments comprise a variety of therapeutic modalities intended to offer patients more precise and potent relief. Regenerative medicine is one prominent field of study, where the application of growth factors and stem cells shows promise for fostering tissue regeneration and repair in the damaged spinal segments. Researchers are looking into how regenerative therapies can help people with spondylolisthesis mend more quickly and have better overall results.

Furthermore, there have been notable advancements in the field of minimally invasive methods when it comes to treating spondylolisthesis. Patients heal more quickly and have less pain after surgery thanks to these treatments' smaller incisions and decreased tissue disruption. As a feasible alternative for treating spondylolisthesis, minimally invasive spine surgery is becoming more and more well-liked since it strikes a balance between patient-friendly care and successful intervention.

ADVANCES IN THE TREATMENT OF SPONDYLOLISTHESIS

Advances in the management of spondylolisthesis care go beyond specific treatment techniques and include a whole-person approach to patient care. To maximize results, holistic approaches now include improvements in patient education, tailored treatment regimens, and diagnostic technologies. Advanced MRI and CT scans are examples of diagnostic imaging tools that offer thorough insights into the amount and nature of spondylolisthesis, allowing medical personnel to more accurately adapt treatment plans.

Moreover, interdisciplinary care models—which entail cooperation between orthopedic surgeons, neurologists, physiotherapists, and pain management specialists— are becoming more and more popular. This team approach guarantees that patients receive a comprehensive and well-coordinated continuum of therapy that addresses the psychological and social aspects of spondylolisthesis in addition to its clinical manifestations.

CLINICAL TRIALS AND RESEARCH INITIATIVES

Research projects and clinical trials are essential for expanding our knowledge of spondylolisthesis and improving our methods of therapy. Current research investigates new therapeutic approaches, assesses the long-term effectiveness of current treatments, and helps to create evidence-based guidelines for the management of spondylolisthesis. Large-scale partnerships involving academic institutions, healthcare providers, and business partners are a part of these programs.

Testing the efficacy and safety of novel therapies and technologies requires the use of clinical trials. In these trials, patients provide important information that helps doctors and researchers understand how interventions work in the real world. Furthermore, as a more thorough understanding of the condition informs treatment decisions, longitudinal studies are providing light on the natural history of spondylolisthesis and aiding in the identification of risk factors and the improvement of diagnostic criteria.